SEE

SAW

(A Memoir)

By: Vernetta Norman

John 9:5-7 vs

While I am in the world, I am the
light of the world."

[6] After saying this, he spit on the
ground, made some mud with the
saliva, and put it on the man's eyes.
[7] "Go," he told him, "wash in the Pool
of Siloam" (this word means "Sent").
So the man went and washed, and
came home seeing.

Dedication

To some that have visual conditions;
and those whom are not aware of
having a visual condition.

It's What I Experience

1990

"Come here a minute, please. There seems to be something in my eye!" I summoned my three children.

"Oh, my goodness. Mom, what is that in your left eye" Asked my one son and two daughters.'

It feels like something very sharp has gotten into my eye; like glass. In which I know is impossible. What discomfort it's causing. I'll call to make an appointment with my Ophthalmologist to check it out.

"Yeah, Mom we don't want you to ignore that. You need your eyes." The children stated.

I got an immediate appointment to see an eye specialist.

Following extensive eye exams for many months. Which turned into years? Finally In 1996. I left my eye appointment very disappointed; totally devastated at the findings.

Many other specialists were called in weeks later to my surprise, they found the eye issue. What I called "bumps" in my eye, is actually called…..

"Pterygium"

The specialists called it "Pterygium" (conjunctiva) pronounced (tuh-RIJ-ee-uhm) is an elevated, wedged-shaped bump on the eyeball that starts on the white of the eye (sclera) and can invade the cornea. The specialists believe that this type of eye disease come from serious "dry eyes." Some

specialists call the "Pterygium"
surfers eyes.

 I called it an attack of my eye that I
really needed, to accomplish my goal.
After all, for years I had finally
prepared special timing to attend
Nursing School to become a
Registered Nurse Practitioner. A
longtime dream of mine. Now, odds
are against me? What?

Lord, this cannot be happening to me.
I need your help with this serious
matter. At least to me it was not
happening.

Years have passed and this irritating
eye condition lingers; it's devastating
attack remains unpredictable.

While every day is a huge challenge
for me, I began to explore my options.
Would I continue to not fulfill my
dreams, or would I live my dreams
with determination.

I've pondered with this question for so long due to being legally blind in my left eye, with low vision in my right eye. My conclusion shocked even me. I decided to ...."Soar Like An Eagle."

I began to ignore those dead medical-dilemmas of what I cannot accomplish; of shaking of their heads or, "We're so sorry there's nothing we can do; you can live with this. Or, we can remove the Pterygium again, but it will probably come back.

Phooey, with the dumb talk. Why would I even contemplate risking more damage to my eye? Life experiences will teach all of us that no matter the condition we must make a godly decision for our own satisfaction. While making a decisive decision. I am still in dismay today, extremely disappointed and reminded daily when I do a close-up of the unsightly remaining eye scaring.

All of the stress from this eye condition is in an enormous state. People might assume that I'm frowning or angry about something; when actually the eye discomfort places me in an uncomforting position. Pressure builds up in both eyes, which causes my eyes to not relax. Restlessness becomes a daily and nightly routine. Tossing and pacing the floor is overwhelming at times. I ask myself, and then I ask my God, when will this situation get better.

To no avail, I have no answer. So, I tarry on, trusting that something will brake for the good. Hopefully I will get the solid answer one day. Whether it's a sunny or cloudy day, I wear my eye-gear daily to protect my eyes from the light of the sun-rays. Oh, yes, even on a cloudy day my eyes disagree with the light.

Change Has Come

I've learned to complete my tasks in a far different manner now days. Actually, since the diagnosis of having "Pterygium" in 1996, I've developed great skills; better than ever. As far as my personal grooming; I'm extremely more attentive. Everything has to be exact; my hair is well cared for, always intact. My attire remains a crucial element in my daily life. I always loved to dress well, but now, I must be certain that all of my clothing are matching in color and are on the right side.

On several occasions after I have bathed, got fully dressed, looking good; later I find that my top is on the wrong side! I thank God up above that I had on a jacket and no one knew my secret.

Those of us dealing with low vision, blindness or legally blind find these types of "good days" to be rather humorous. We began to have much to laugh about. I know that I do!

While in the kitchen, one must be very cautious. It's essential to always separate the utensils, glassware, pots and pans in their designated places. It's best to have in mind exactly what you want to prepare. Know your way around so that you or anyone else doesn't stumble; at least not too much stumbling. I don't accidently leave the stove on, any more. My explanation is plain; you can start a fire! Therefore, be sure to turn the stove off; then double check to be sure that it's off. I learn to not cook, and then leave the area; it's not a smart thing to do.

Sometimes, I call myself multitasking. This is a really bad idea. I get occupied with what I'm doing in another room; then it hit me to check my food. So, I'm racing to quickly investigate my damage. Luckily, God allowed me to catch it in time, to eliminate a catastrophe. The bathroom can be a danger as well if you don't set things in their proper place. I'm not one to leave things lying around and I never leave water running. Besides who wants to clean up the mess.

Outside

Since I think that I understand the nature of Pterygium, I had a habit of not wanting to be alone outside by myself. This is true fact.

Years back, I had to ride public transportation. I prayed to aboard the correct bus to my destination. When I a boarded the bus, I had the nerve to pay far more than my fare. I knew this, because each person that boarded the bus after I did didn't have to pay. People start saying, "I wish she'd give me some of that money."

Suddenly, it hit me…….Girl, you put in a good piece of money into that slot. Sure enough after I got to a designated place, I double checked my purse. You guessed right! Instead of placing $2.25 in the slot, I put my $10.00 bill in that darn slot.

Lord, I don't have that to spare, not today, I thought to myself. What should I do? Should I call the bus terminal? I need my money back, like now, today. Then, I solved my issue and thought. I saw a lot of elderly board that bus and they could have not had much money either.

I concluded that apparently God meant for me to be a blessing to strangers that day. So, I sowed that seed honorably

Have a Heart

I realized that my surroundings meant everything. When going through this life and something comes along, basically tare you down. Don't back into a corner to give up. You must grab on to the life God provided you, and then get up!

It took a while for me to grab this concept, but I eventually got the message.

I was already in a position to not ever have a pity-party for myself. I knew that I'm too independent for that. I began to occupy my mind with good thoughts. Yet in the back of my mind were thoughts of –sistah, are you ready for this? Why me?

Understand, it's not easy living with Pterygium, nor is it the end either. I self-taught "myself" on what to and not to allow in my spirit. I again found out what works for me so that I can enjoy everyday life. After all, if you think negative about yourself, others will have no need to think any different of you. Don't be a bore; stay positive as much as possible.

There are many days which seem like things are going up and down, twisted. I pray it away and engaged with family and others who make me stronger in mind and spirit. The essence of life is to help others who may be dealing with the same issue that you're encountering. When I inform others to push-on regardless of their situation, I feel like I've accomplished a lot. T realize that someone is being healed and comforted is rewarding to me. I have met people with different types of situations who only needed that assurance that they will recover from what ails them. I call it having compassion; a concern to help others live a normal life in- spite-of.

Awww, what a blessed feeling it is to "pass-the-baton" of a gift giving life to another hurting person, so they may live.

These thoughts pop up now and then, but I've moved on. My intent is to globally speak at, schools, universities, churches, clinics, hospitals and anywhere to educate others and their families about Pterygium.

I am determined to follow my dream, which is to start my own "IPOP'N Foundation" very soon. There continues to be known fact that research is unending. I must dedicate my timely efforts to assure others that a cure for "Pterygium" will eventually come.

Healthy Notes

I've always believed in having excellent healthy intake, following my

"Rules-of-Thumb"

1. Health food and beverage intake is vital. Consuming fresh veggies, especially carrots, leafy greens and fruits

2. Drink "Clean" Water

3. Moderate exercise

4. Lots of Laughter

Protect Your Eyes

Be extremely careful of getting tap water into your eyes because the chlorine will "burn" them. Sterile eye drops (water) is a must, but be very cautious of the brands of (bottled) water.

A saying is, "Everything" that looks good is not necessarily good for you." I state this because some bottled water is actually "tap."

My eyes are extremely sensitive to light, tv, reading and my list goes on and on. Therefore, I found that I cannot use any type of water(s) or eye drop. I have to use a "top-of-the-line eye moisture product. Yes, with "Pterygium," using a top brand of eye product is critical. The "Pterygium" is growth and the only thing that I want for my body and yours is ...."Good Health."

Like our bodies, as we get older we have to moisturize it. The same rule is evident to have healthy eyes. I was given

prescription eye drops to moisturize me eyes; in which agitated them. Again, I researched on my own and found an eye moisturizer that works for my eyes! Moisturizing my eyes help to stop the unsightly grow of the "Pterygium." Find the right one for "you" and keep your eyes…

HEALTHY and "MOISTURIZED"

The "SEESAW's" in this life come only to motivate your faith. Giving you strength to endure, to conquer. Be worry free, and then receive the blessing. Whatever the issue, don't fall off. Stay balanced!

Be Encouraged; Be Blessed above all….Be Happy!!!!

SEESAW

One day I looked over yonder and
what did I see

I looked in my mirror, I could barely
see me.

My face was basically in a blur,

I panicked and thought,

What can this be?

In attempt to stretch my eyes- to get a
good view,

All I could notice was that cloudiness
had intervened-

It was not a time to scream.

While I didn't get an immediate
answer,

I fell to my knees in Prayer….

I asked The LORD to ….

Help me please!

It took some time, but He heard my cry,

The Lord replied," Child, nothings too hard for me. You're already healed…

Know your rightful place in life,

I want you to help others who have something far worst.

You only have to …BELIEVE!

So, now, my daughter…

You can……. "C"

www.ingramcontent.com/pod-product-compliance
Lightning Source LLC
Chambersburg PA
CBHW021347310526
45786CB00020B/2001